YOUR KNOWLEDGE HAS VALUE

- We will publish your bachelor's and
  master's thesis, essays and papers

- Your own eBook and book -
  sold worldwide in all relevant shops

- Earn money with each sale

Upload your text at www.GRIN.com
and publish for free

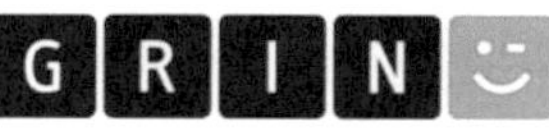

Kingsley Adimabua, A. M. Odiegwu, G. A. Awemu

A Systematic Review of the Causal Link between Stress and Hypertension with the Use of Hills Criteria of Causation

GRIN Publishing

Bibliographic information published by the German National Library:

The German National Library lists this publication in the National Bibliography;
detailed bibliographic data are available on the Internet at http://dnb.dnb.de .

Imprint:

Copyright © 2013 GRIN Verlag, Open Publishing GmbH
Print and binding: Books on Demand GmbH, Norderstedt Germany
ISBN: 978-3-656-92867-6

This book at GRIN:

http://www.grin.com/en/e-book/207814/a-systematic-review-of-the-causal-link-
between-stress-and-hypertension

A Systematic Review of the Causal link between stress and hypertension with the use of Hills Criteria of Causation

A.M. Odiegwu[1], K.O. Adimabua[2], G. A. Awemu[3]

[1]Department of Nursing Science, Madonna University, Elele, Nigeria

[2]Department of Public Health, Madonna University, Elele, Nigeria

[3]Department of Pharmaceutical and Medicinal Chemistry, Madonna University, Elele, Nigeria

Abstract

Background context

There is little or no doubt that stressful situations can cause significant rise in blood pressure. It is no news that a more chronic form of blood pressure is termed "hypertension". There is a need to discover whether the presence of stress really leads to the development over time.

Study Design

A systematic review of literature on stress and hypertension

Sample

Studies reporting an association between stress and hypertension

Methods

A systematic review was carried out to identify, evaluate and summarize the literature related to establishing a causal relationship between stress and hypertension with the use of Bradford-Hills criteria of causality. A search was carried out using CINAHL, MEDLINE, and Pub Med databases and their reference list of included study and other internet sources Keywords like stress, hypertension, plausibility, dose-response relationship, temporality, coherence, analogy, and epidemiology was used as the search criteria.

Results

The search yielded 10 studies with about 2,000 citations. 4 studies provided moderate evidence for the causation criterion and 6 studies provided strong evidence for the causal criterion. None of the studies agreed with specificity of causes as a criterion for determining that stress causes hypertensions and no study was found that suggests analogy between stress and hypertension

Conclusion

There is enough significant evidence to fulfill the basic criteria of causation as proposed by Austin Bradford Hill.

Introduction

In 1843, John Stuart Mill wrote a book titled *"A System of Logic: Ratiocination and Induction."* This text was used to judge causal relationships through the following means: method of agreement, method of difference, joint method of agreement and difference, method residues, and method of concomitant variation (Dishman, Washburn, and Heath: 2004). During that period this was the basic tool used to determine causation between two variables. Not until 1965 when Sir Austin Bradford Hill (Hill, 1965) developed another causation criteria that is used till this very day. His proposed criteria included the following criterion, Consistency, Dose Response Relationship, Temporality, Coherence, Theoretical Plausibility, Experimental Evidence, Specificity, Strength of Association and Analogy. They form the fundamental prerequisites and assessment criteria of the cause-effect relationship (Jenicek, 2004)

Hill's criteria apply to stress and hypertension because of several arguments that suggests that stress cause or do not cause hypertension. Many argue that there is little doubt that both physical and mental stress can cause significant elevations of high blood pressure. But long term exposure to high blood pressure is hypertension. So can stress play a role in development of hypertension?

It will be useful to define each of the 9 criteria which are Analogy, Coherence, Theoretical plausibility, Dose response relationship, Experimental evidence, Consistency, Strength of association, Specificity and Temporality.

Table 1: Hill's Criteria Definitions

CRITERION	DEFINITION
Consistency	An association between cause and effect should be robust enough to be demonstrable in multiple studies by different investigators (Hill, 1965). This is key to understanding the fallacy of presenting a single study as definitive evidence for or against a disease etiology or treatment effect.
Dose response relationship	There should be a direct relationship between the risk factor (i.e., the independent variable) and people's status on the disease variable (i.e., the dependent variable)
Specificity	If a putative cause is associated with a very specific set of symptoms, or a treatment with very specific effects, this supports a causal relationship. If the cause is present with a wide variety of different clinical presentations or the results following a treatment are highly variable, this argues against a causal relationship (Hill, 1965)
Temporality	Causes by definition precede their effects, so if a potential causal agent is observed after the condition it is speculated to be causing, this argues strongly against a true etiologic relationship (Hill, 1965)
Strength of Association	The strength of an association can be supportive of a true underlying causal relationship. If a proposed cause for a disease is associated with the disease itself only sporadically or unpredictably, this is weaker evidence for its causal role than if it is reliably present in conjunction with the disease. (Hill, 1965)
Theoretical Plausibility	It is easier to accept an association as causal when there is a rational and theoretical basis for such a conclusion
Experimental Evidence	Any related research that is based on experiments will make a

	causal inference more plausible
Coherence	A cause-and-effect interpretation for an association is clearest when it does not conflict with what is known about the variables under study and when there are no plausible competing theories or rival hypotheses. In other words, the association must be coherent with other knowledge.
Analogy	This is perhaps the weakest of Hill's criteria, Sometimes a commonly accepted phenomenon in one area can be applied to another area

Methods

A search was carried out using CINAHL, MEDLINE, and Pub Med databases and their reference list of included study and other internet sources. Keywords like stress, hypertension, plausibility, dose-response relationship, temporality, coherence, analogy, and epidemiology was used as the search criteria. Combinations of the above mentioned words were also used during the search, this was to aid in specific areas of the search. Results from the search that were of no importance were discarded and more key words like blood pressure and mortality in combination with the above mentioned terms yielded the desired search results.

Results

Each of the criteria proposed by Dr. Hill was assessed independently as an individual entity. The result of the literature review was separated by Analogy, Coherence, Theoretical plausibility, Dose response relationship, Experimental evidence, Consistency, Strength of association, Specificity and Temporality. Overall, studies show a satisfactory link between stress and hypertension.

Specificity of causes and analogy was not consistent with the findings of the study

Discussions

The strength of the evidence for concluding that there is a cause and an effect association between two entities must be judged by Hill's Criteria (Dishman, 2004)
If Stress is thought to be a cause, then there must logically be an effect. When a statistical association between a risk factor (e.g., stress) and a disease outcome (e.g., hypertension) can be demonstrated, Hill's Criteria increases the probability that the association is causal (Dishman, Washburn , Heath: 2004). It would seem that this is an accurate assumption when the results of confounding variables and effect modification have been controlled.

Strength of association
Strength is defined as the size of the risk as measured by appropriate statistical tests (Gordis, 2004) and is based on measurement (Colley, Morgan, Haas: 1998). It essentially asks the question "is the disease rate many times greater among an exposed population?" (Jenicek, 2004) In other words, the larger the association, the more likely the exposure is causing the disease (Rothman, 2002).

A spike in blood pressure is a direct result of stress (mayo clinic). often times, people who have stressful situations have hypertension (Anderson, 2007)

John Hall suggested in Hurst's textbook on heart disease that, "Chronic stress may lead to long-term increases in blood pressure (Hypertension). Epidemiologic studies show that air traffic controllers, lower socioeconomic groups and other groups who are believed to have stressful lives, have increased prevalence of hypertension (Kulkarni, 1998)

These findings suggest that there is strength in association between stress and hypertension in relation to a causal link.

Experimental Evidence

Experimental evidence is defined as the condition can be altered (prevented or ameliorated) by an appropriate experimental regimen (Last, 2001). Rothman (2002) argued that, as a criterion, experimental evidence cannot be applied to all settings. However, the one area in which the experimental evidence criterion can be applied to is in the animal model.

In relation to this study, Animal studies support the point of view that stressful situations can lead to high blood pressure which will eventually lead to hypertension. For example, mice develop high blood pressure when crowded in small cages. (Green, Kreuter, 1999). Similar trends are described in dogs and non human primates (Jenicek, 2004) and it is very familiar that the physiologic make up of these animals are very similar to man. The study of overcrowding in mice suggests that people living in dense urban environments should endeavor to visit recreational parks and centers. These study provided experimental evidence in the causal link between stress and hypertension.

Dose Response Relationship

Dose-response is defined as an increasing level of exposure (in amount and/or time) increases the risk (Last, 2001). Dose-response can be approached by asking the question "does the association show a dose response effect i.e. does the more exposure a group of people has proportionately increases the frequency of disease experienced?" (Jenicek, 2004) This criterion is an extension of the strength criterion and is based on measurement (Jenicek, 2004). It can be explained as the measurement of the relationship amount of exposure in duration, intensity, quality and the size of the impact.

In relation to stress and hypertension, increased exposure to stressful situations often result to hypertension over time (Kulkarni, 1998) and this was consistent with other findings in other literature.

Hence it wouldn't be wrong to assume a causal relationship between stress and hypertension based on the Dose Response Relationship.

Specificity in Causes

Specificity reveals that a factor (cause under study) leads to a consistent pattern of consequences (Jenicek, 2004). In other words, a single putative cause should produce a specific effect (Gordis, 2004).

Overall studies show that stress does not directly cause hypertension but can have an effect on its development. Although a single cause may not be identified, the general consensus is that various factors contribute to blood pressure elevation in essential hypertension.

Unhealthy lifestyles can predispose someone to hypertension e.g. overeating, smoking, increased alcohol use, over use of caffeine and poor sleep habits.

This shows that the causal link between stress and hypertension is not specific.

Coherence

Coherence is the association should be compatible with existing theory and knowledge (Last, 2001). The criterion essentially asks the question "is the association supported by generally known facts about the natural history and biology of the disease?" (Jenicek, 2004) To qualify as a study to match the coherence criterion a study would have to have been performed that would have suggested stress as a causal factor of disease and would have to be implicated in a certain disease or pathological state. In other words, in the case of a specific disease would the facts of that disease support the notion that Stress as the causal factor.

Studies were in agreement with this criterion. Hypertension risk factors such as obesity, smoking, excess alcohol intake, and salt intake are heightened when stress is also a factor (Anderson, 2007)

Temporality

Temporal sequence is the only absolutely essential criterion for a cause-effect association (Last, 2001). It asks the question "did the exposure occur before the disease began?" It (temporal sequence) must be clearly defined as the "cart is firmly behind the horse" (Jenicek, 2004). This suggests that stress must always precede hypertension for a true cause and effect scenario to take place. If a stress is present for any period of time, a progression of ill effects should be observed when there is an increase in magnitude over the same period of time. There was temporal sequence between stress and hypertension in the studies reviewed. John Hall (2010) suggested that chronic stress must be present before the onset of hypertension and this was consistent with other literature.

Theoretical Plausibility

It is easier to accept an association as causal when there is a rational and theoretical basis for such a conclusion. Plausibility refers to the coherence with the current of body of biologic knowledge (Gordis, 2004). The association causing an effect must agree with currently accepted understanding of pathobiological processes (Last, 2001). The criterion asks the question "does a pathophysiologic model of how the exposure could cause the disease make sense?"

The theory that stress can alter the way the body normally works seem viable. While at stressful state, the body releases adrenalin and this in turn raises the heart beat rate which eventually may lead to hypertension (Kulkarni, 1998). This was consistent with other findings. Hence, there is theoretical plausibility between stress as a causative factor to hypertension.

Consistency

Consistency pertains to the association being noted consistently, across many studies in different people, places and circumstances and times (Jenicek, 2004). Results need to be replicated in many studies.

Kulkarni (1998) suggests in his article "Stress and Hypertension" That. There is a consistent relationship between stress and hypertension He discovered that almost all the cases he studied for stress had hypertension this was also consistent with the findings from the American Institute for Stress. Their results were still consistent with both sexes and people of all races.

Analogy

The analogy criterion looks for a disease or exposure that may have been observed that may be of similarity. It essentially asks the question if there are no other epidemiologic or experimental studies of this exposure-disease relationship, has a causal association been established for a very similar agent. (Jenicek, 2004) No studies were found that offered a consistent analogy linking between stress and hypertension.

Table 2: Hill's Criteria of Causation Applied to Stress and Hypertension

Criteria	Result
Strength	All Studies Showed strength of association in the causal ilnk between stress and hypertension
Specificity	Studies did not indicate speciticity in causes between stress and hypertension
Consistency	There was consistency in the causal link between stress and hypertension
Temporality	Studies showed temporality between stress and hypertension
Experimental Evidence	Studies showed a causal link between stress and hypertension with sufficient experimental evidence
Dose Response Relationship	There was a link in dose and response relationship i.e. biological gradient between stress and hypertension
Theoretical Plausibility	There was evidence of theoretical Plausibility
Coherence	The causal link between stress and hypertension was coherent with already known knowledge from the literature reviewed
Analogy	No studies were found that suggested coherence between stress and hypertension

Limitations to utilizing Hill's Criteria

Hill's Criteria do have some limitations. The only criterion of Hill's that is truly a causal criterion is temporality while suggesting that the other criteria were vague (Rothman, 2002). Although these criteria were never designed to be hard and fast rules, they do provide essential guidelines for establishing causation (Lucas and McMichael, 2005). Nevertheless, the criteria of Hill remain as basic principles in finding causal relationships. Henneken and Buring's criteria are better due to the incorporation of statistical concepts and de-emphasizes the weaker criterion of analogy (Henneken and Buring, 1987). Nevertheless, if a concept such as Stress and hypertension fails the test established by Hill's Criteria, it would seem that the application of Henneken and Buring's criteria is premature. Phillips and Goodman (2004) have noted, in relation to Hill's criteria, that statistical significance should not be mistaken for evidence of a substantial association, association does not prove causation (other evidence must be considered), precision should not be mistaken for validity (non-random errors exist), and uncertainty about whether there is a causal relationship (or even an association) is not sufficient to suggest action should not be taken. However, these same authors noted that evidence (or belief) that there is a causal relationship is not sufficient to suggest action should be taken (Phillips and Goodman, 2004).

Conclusion

There is significant evidence in the literature to fulfill Hill's criteria of causation with regards to stress as a causative agent to hypertension.

REFERENCES

1. Dishman RK, Washburn RA, Heath GW: **Physical Activity Epidemiology.** Human Kinetics. Champaign, IL; 2004.
2. Hill AB: **The environment and disease: association or causation?** *Proc R Soc Med* 1965, **58:**295-300.
3. Jenicek M: **Foundations of Evidence-Based Medicine.** Partheon Publishing. Boca Raton; 2004.
4. Keating JC: **Letter: Evaluating the quality of clinical practice guidelines.** *J Manipulative Physiol Ther* 2003, **26(3):**1-4.
5. Keating JC: **Philosophy: the art of skepticism.** *J Can Chiropr Assoc* 2000, **44(2):**79-84.
6. Plaugher G, Long CR, Alcantara K, Silveus A, Wood H, Lotun K, Menke M, Meeker WC, Rowe SH: **Practice-based randomized controlled-comparison clinical trial of chiropractic adjustments and brief massage treatment at sites of subluxation in subjects with essential hypertension: pilot study.** *J Manipulative Physiol Ther* 2002, **25:**221-239.
7. Keating JC, Hyde TE, Menke JM, Seaman D, Vincent RE, Wyatt LH: **In the quest for cultural authority.** *Dyn Chiro* 2004, **26(22):**1-2.
8. Green LW, Kreuter MW: **Health Promotion Planning: An Educational and Ecological Approach.** Third edition. Mayfield Publishing Company. Mountain View, California; 1999.
9. Colley F, Morgan L, Haas M: **Reply to "issues" in chiropractic pediatrics: vaccination.** *Dyn Chiro* 1998, **16(9):**.
10. Rothman KJ: **Epidemiology: An Introduction.** Oxford University Press. New York, NY; 2002.
11. Last JM: **A Dictionary of Epidemiology.** 4th edition. Oxford University Press. New York, NY; 2001.
12. Gordis L: **Epidemiology.** 3rd edition. Elsevier Saunders. Philadelphia. PA; 2004.
13. Biggs L, Mierau D, Hay D: **Measuring philosophy: a philosophy index.** *J Can Chiropr Assoc* 2002, **46(3):**173-183.
14. Meeker WC: **Teaching skills that fit the needs of the clinician: an argument for the role of clinical epidemiology in teaching evidence-based practice.** *WFC/ACC/NBCE: Innovations and Challenges in Clinical Education* 2002.
15. McCoy M: **Telling Time the truth.** *The Chiro J* 2001.
16. Mootz RD, Shekelle PG, Hansen DT: **The politics of policy and research.** *Topics Clin Chiro* 1995, **2(2):**56-70.
17. Lucas RM, McMichael AJ: **Association or causation: evaluating links between "environment and disease".** *Bull World Health Organ* 2005, **83(10):**792-795.
18. Henneken CH, Buring JE: **Epidemiology in Medicine.** Edited by: Mayrent SL. Little, Brown and Company. Boston; 1987.
19. Phillips CV, Goodman KJ: **The mixed lessons of Sir Austin Bradford Hill.** *Epidemiol Perspect Innov* 2004, **1:**1-5.
20. Kulkarni S. **Stress and Hypertension** *wmj.* 1998. *Medical Colllege of Wisconsin.* Milwaukee USA
21. Stress and High blood pressure, retrieved from www.mayoclinic.com: July 2012
22. Stress retrieved from www.stress.org/topic-hypertension.htm: July 2012